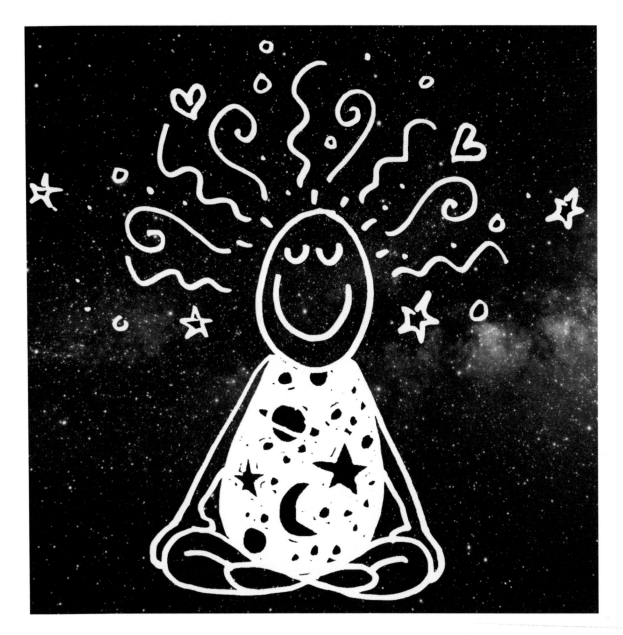

I am the UNIVERSE

I am the UNIVERSE!

DEDICATION

To the Universe, and every single thing it has disguised itself to be.

Yoga is a beautiful practice to do alone, in class, with friends and with children. We begin to see that although we have many things that separate us in our communities, countries, world… it might not even feel like we belong to the same planet sometimes, we are, most certainly, all in and of the same universe. Happy practicing x

CONTENTS

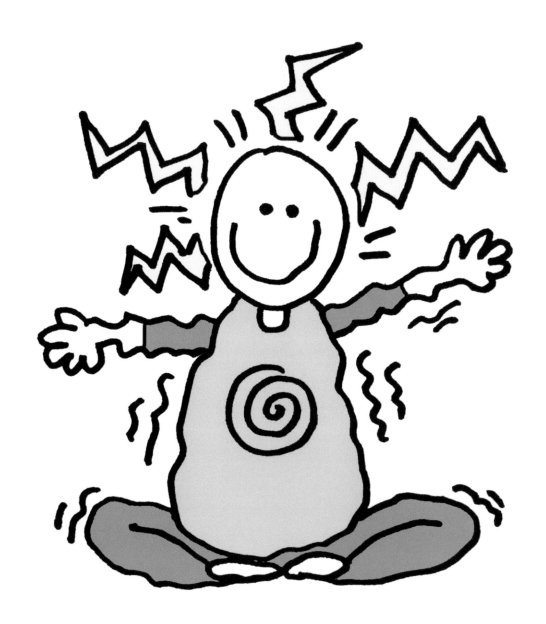

I am ENERGY - I wiggle everywhere! I am made of electricity that wiggles through everything.

I can wiggle high, I can wiggle low. Where can your wiggly energy go?

(Wiggles warm up)

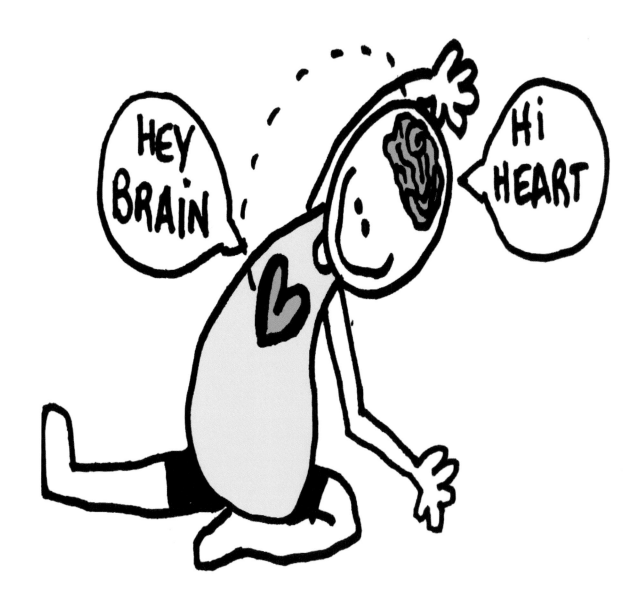

I am PARTICLES – I am a BODY made of particles and energy. I can bend in lots of directions. I am a very special body because my heart and my brain can speak to each other.

(Bending & warming up)

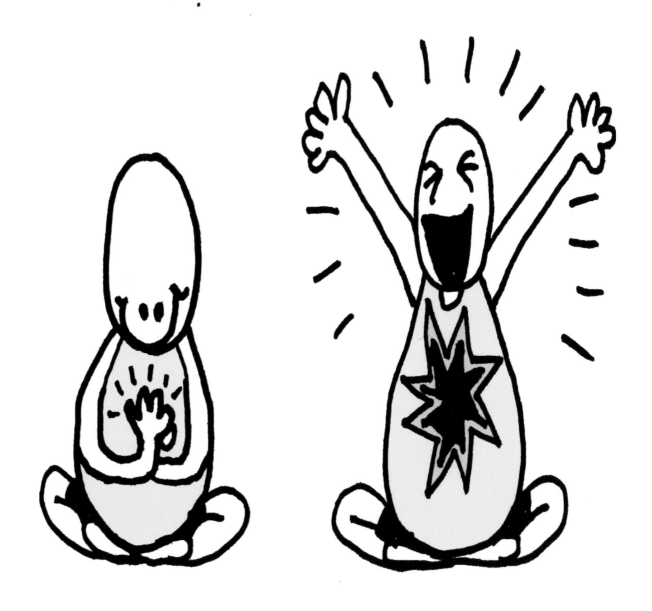

I am a BIG BANG – First, I twinkle like a star and get so hot that I explode! There is a lot of sound and light.

How loud and soft can you make your Big Bang?

(Twinkle small & stretch big)

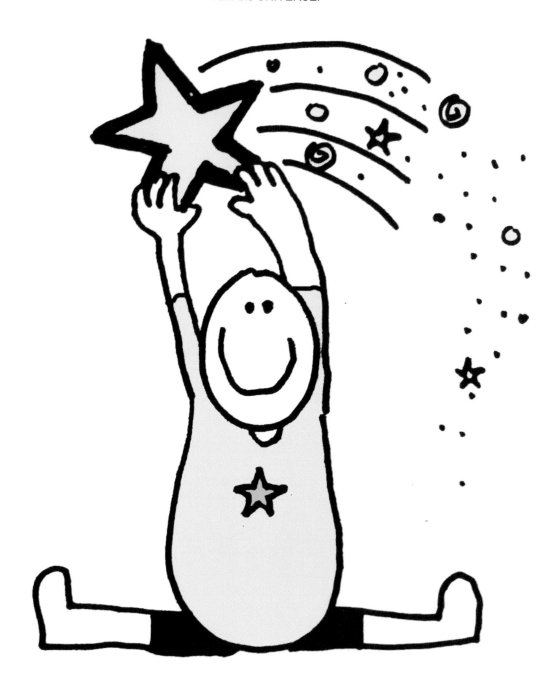

I am STARDUST - Stardust made the Milky Way galaxy. I am shooting stars with paths of glitter. I zoom across the night sky. What is your wish today?

(Shooting Star with breath)

I am the UNIVERSE!

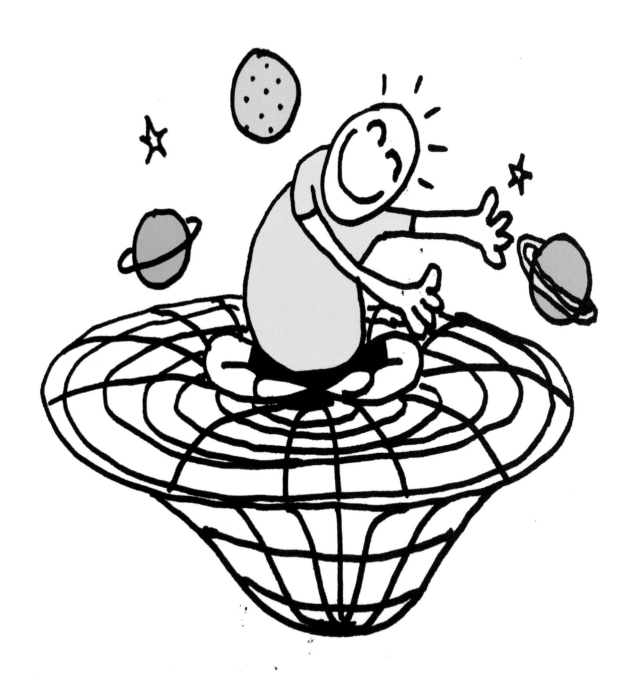

I am the PLANETS - I bend Space-Time this way and that. I whizz round and round the sun in a spinning orbit. What colour is your planet?

(Rotation work. Running in circles. Working with gravity)

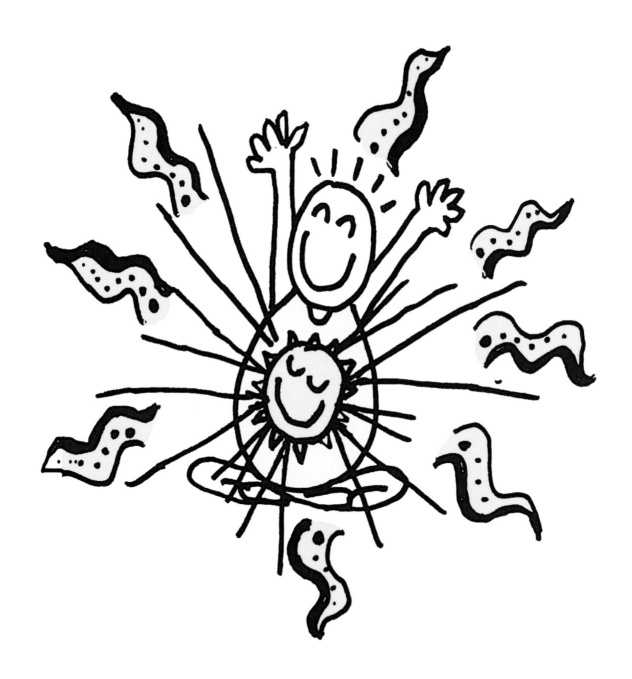

I am the SUN - I give life to everything. I share my light, kindness and love for free!

(Sun Salutations)

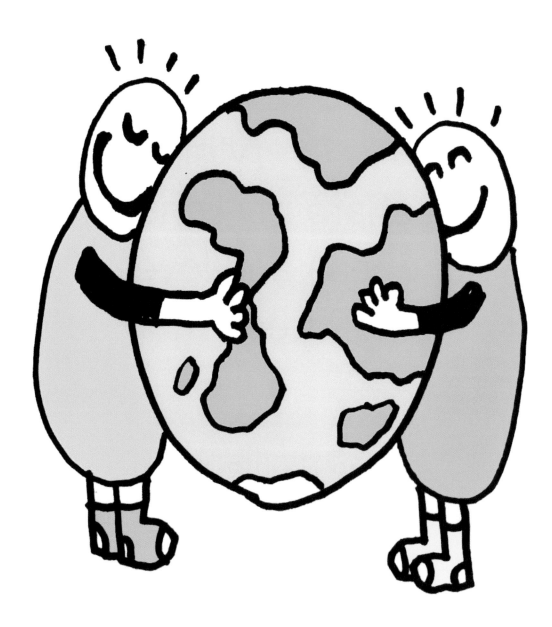

I am PLANET EARTH -
When I hug myself, I
give the world a big hug.
I am my own home and
the world is my home.
What do you love about
Planet Earth?

(Big Hug, Spine relaxing)

I am the UNIVERSE!

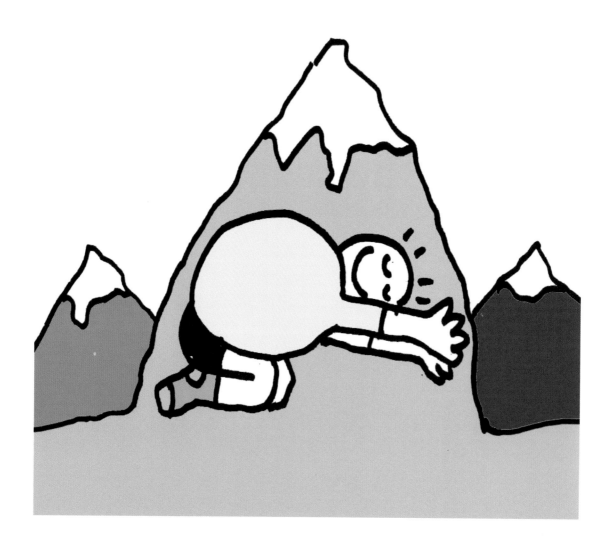

I am a ROCK - Whenever I need to rest or feel grounded, I curl up and stay still. I feel relaxed in my body and I breathe patiently.

(Child's Pose)

I am the UNIVERSE!

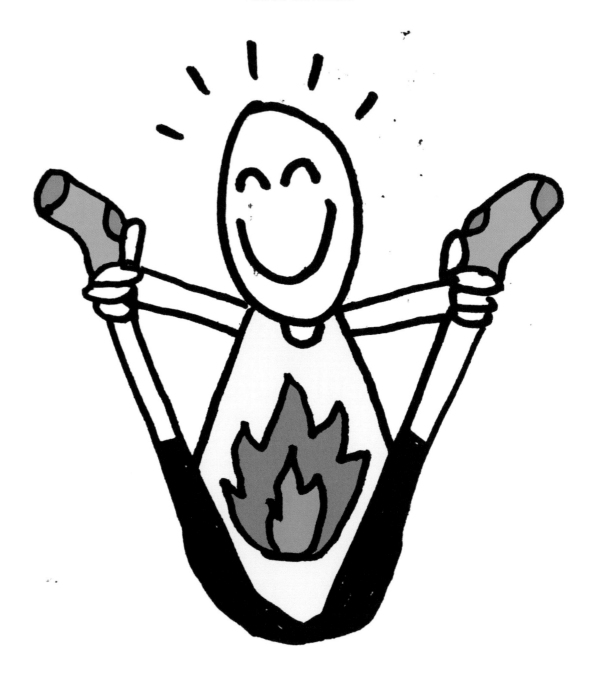

I am FIRE - At the center of the earth. My core is made of Lava, it is hot and powerful - I sizzle and hiss (Kapalbhati). Sometimes I move, then I am still. What shape do you want to hold today?

(Planks. Core work)

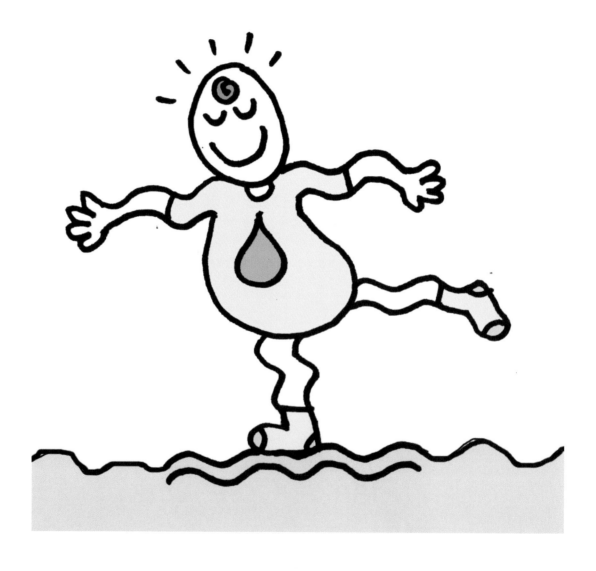

I am WATER - Flowing everywhere. There are no pauses in my movement and my breath sounds like the ocean waves. (Ujjayi breath). When I focus on one thing, my energy flows there like a river. What will you focus on?

(Yoga flows)

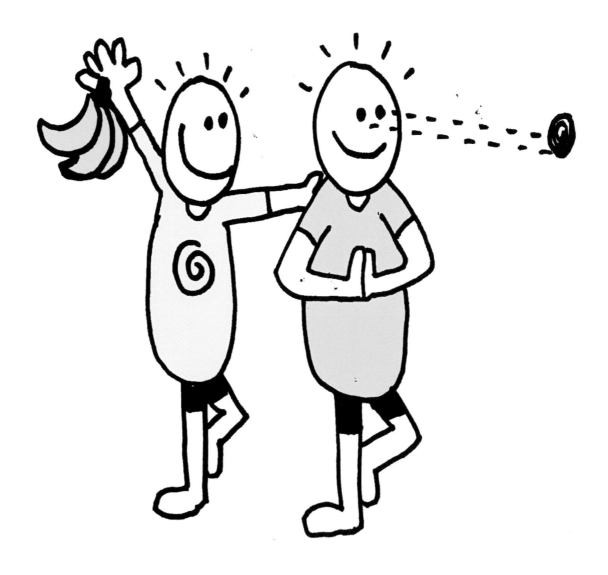

I am a TREE - I stand calm and balanced. I fix my eyes on one point (A Drishti). The wind blows, but I don't fall. Sometimes, I lean on others for support. My branches grow lots of different fruits! What fruit is on your tree?

(Tree pose)

I am the UNIVERSE!

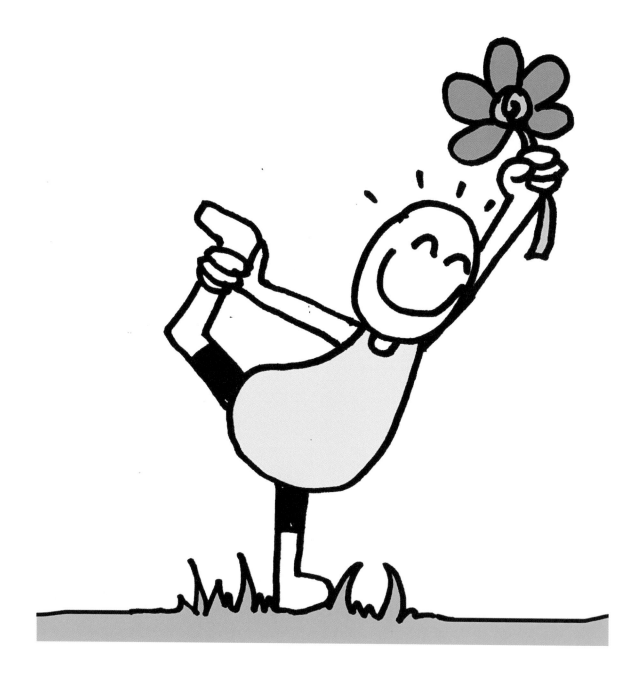

I am a FLOWER - I am beautiful and unique, I bring joy to others. I need light, food, water and big breaths to stay healthy. What flower are you?

(Chair pose, dancers pose, growing like a flower)

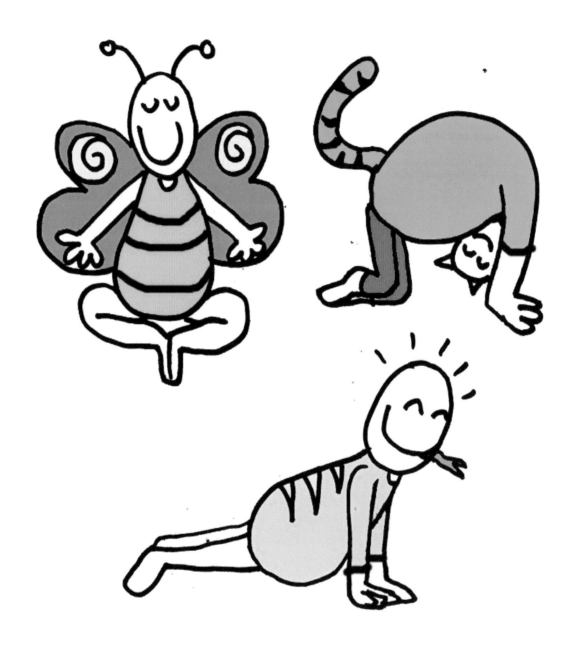

I am the ANIMALS - I can slither like a snake, fly like a crow, stretch like a cat, growl like a tiger, hide like a turtle, wait like a lizard, swim like a fish, flutter like a butterfly... What animal do you like to be?

(Animal postures)

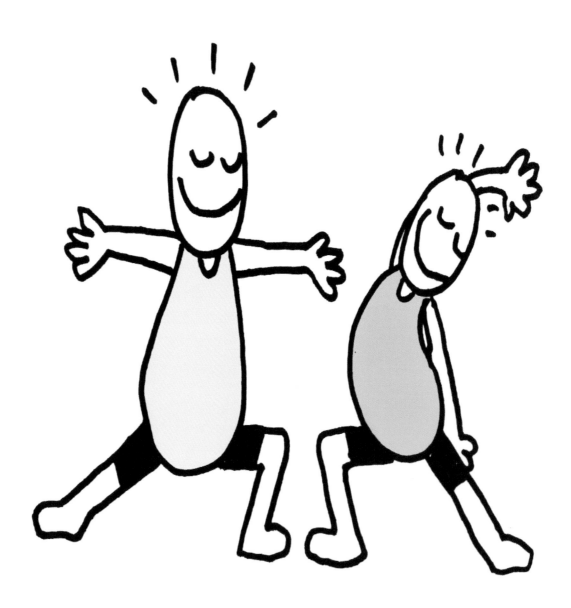

I am a WARRIOR - I am strong and steady, I am ready! I am brave and true. I share my strength with others. How can you be brave?

(Warrior poses)

I am the UNIVERSE!

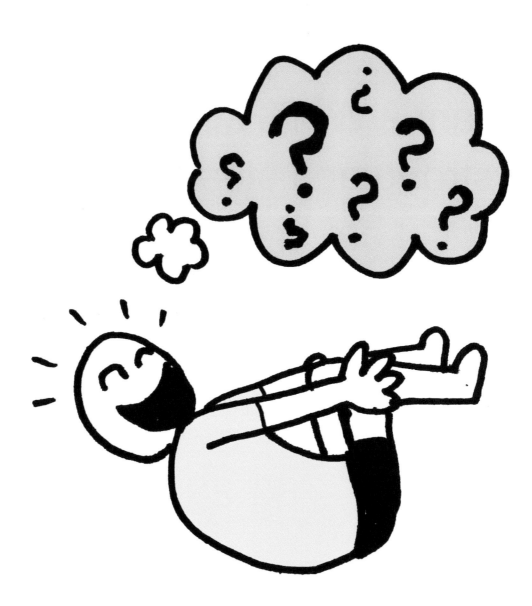

I am a HAPPY BABY - Excited, joyful and very curious. I have lots to learn about the wonderful world! What do you want to learn today?

(Happy baby, Rock and Roll)

I am the UNIVERSE!

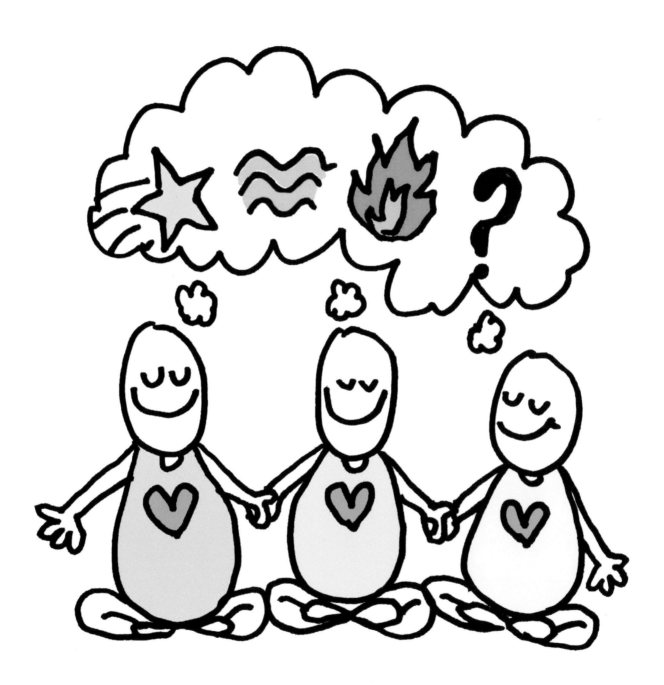

I am a HUMAN - I am very special because I can change my future! All I need is a wish on a star, the focus of a river, the strength of fire, curiosity, hard work and lots of love! How do you want to help other humans?

(Partner work)

I am the UNIVERSE!

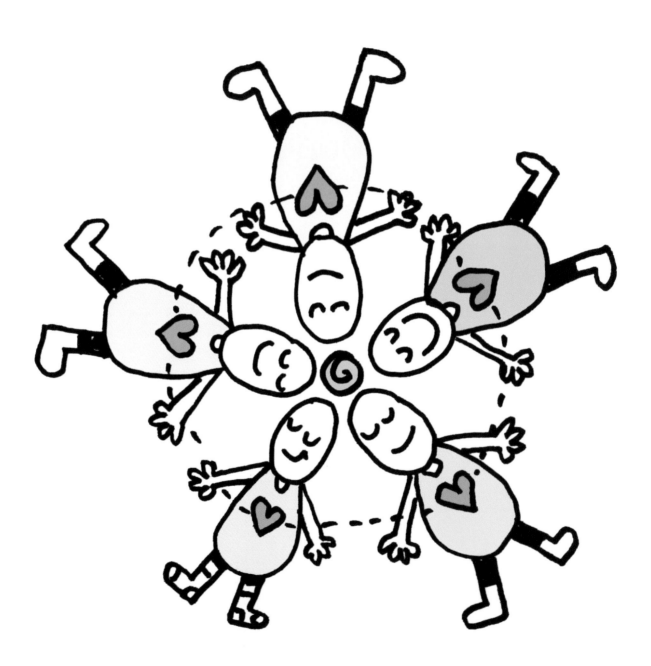

I am EVERYONE! - When I close my eyes and relax my body, I see with my heart. All hearts are the same; they shine like beautiful stars in the night sky and connect with the hearts of others.

(Sivasana)

I am the UNIVERSE!

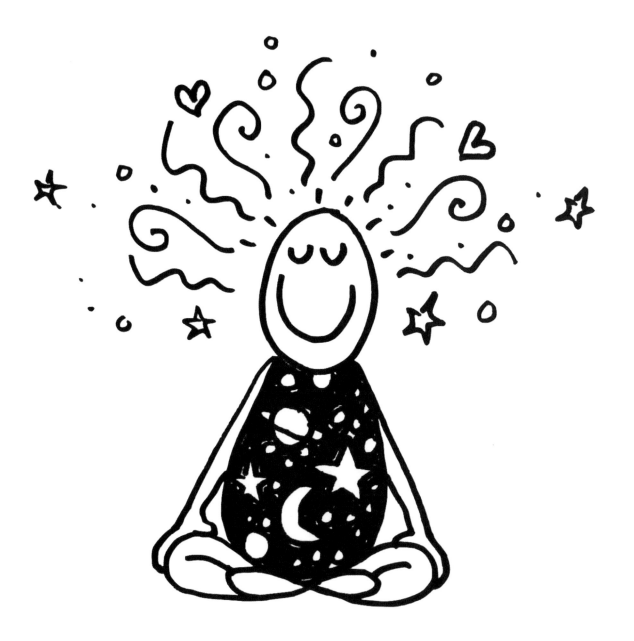

I am the Whole UNIVERSE! - When I breathe in, I breathe as the universe and when I breathe out, my heart glows brighter, lighting up space.

I am unlimited potential…

Ohm, Namaste. The UNIVERSE in me, honors the UNIVERSE in you.

Helpful Glossary:

Ujjayi Breath	A yogic breathing technique of gently constricting the throat so that the breath is more audible and therefore more helpful as a focal point.
Kapalbhati	Shining head! A Pranayama (breathing technique) of short, sharp exhales of breath through the nose and a fast recoil inhale in between each.
Drishti Point	(Pronounced Drish–tee.) A stable, fixed point on which you can focus when in a balancing posture. As your yoga practice deepens you can develop an internal Drishti for balance with closed eyes.

Sivasana	The beautiful relaxation at the end of a yoga class. For this posture, make sure the students are comfortable and warm and the lower back is touching the floor or is very close. Talk through relaxing each limb from the feet to the head.
Sun Salutations	Sun Salutations are a series of postures that give thanks for the sun. The postures, different variations and accompanying Mantras can be found online if you want to add this into a practice at home or in the classroom.

"I am the UNIVERSE!"

Yoga Class:

Energy	**Wiggles Warm up**	Centering: Sitting in a comfortable position, we use our breath to inhale and exhale deeply through the nose. Inhaling energy, growing tall through the spine, and exhaling we send the energy through the body. Sitting or standing, we make the body warm by moving and wiggling it in different ways. You can also play this like a game of musical statues!
Particles	**Body stretch and joint Warm Up**	We bend our particle bodies to gently prepare them for the ASANA (posture) practice. Bending or rotating the neck and head, shoulders, wrists, ankles, knees, hips and then taking a 6 direction back warm up: folding forward, then moving side to side, bending backward and twisting right and left.

Big Bang	**Open Heart**	Breath with shoulder warm ups. Sitting in easy pose. Exhaling: rounding the spine and taking the chin and hands to the chest or hugging the body. Inhaling: opening the arms and chest like a big explosion. Repeat.
Star Dust	**Shoulders**	Hands in Salutation (palms together) at heart center. Inhaling: taking the hands up overhead like a shooting star, Exhaling: Lowering the hands back to the chest. Repeating the movement.
Planets	**Rotations**	1. Warming up fully in preparation for sun salutations. Standing and taking the legs out wide for a straddle. Inhaling: stretching the arms out so we look like a star. Exhaling: taking the body and the arms over to the right and down, making a big circle. Inhaling coming up on the left side. After a few rotations, reversing the direction. 2. Twisting the torso from side to side. Exhaling: rotating round to the right side and looking over the right shoulder. Inhaling: coming back through the center. Exhaling: over to the left side. Repeat.

Sun **Sun Saluta-tions** Giving thanks to the sun. Below is the sequence with the breaths to take with each posture. During sun salutations we stretch and strengthen our body and work with our breath to flow through the sequence. We feel grateful for the light and heat from the sun.

SUN SALUTATIONS – THANK YOU SUN!!

Earth	**Big hug**	Either staying standing or coming down to sitting, we give ourselves a big hug, opening up the back and shoulders and taking big deep breaths into the chest.
Rock	**Childs Pose**	Sitting on the knees and bringing the bottom back towards the heels. The toes are un-tucked and the head comes down to the mat. Arms can stretch out in front (active) or come to the side of the body (passive). We breathe slowly here and relax the shoulders, feeling still and strong like a rock.
Fire	**Core Strength**	Holding core strength postures for a longer time. We can use the pranayama (Yogic Breathing Technique) of **Kapalbhati – Breath of Fire:** short sharp breaths out of the nose, to concentrate and engage the diaphragm to strengthen the abdominals. Postures that are fun to try here are: Boat, spinal column, high, low and side plank, dolphin, side angle, crow, camel.

Water	**Flows**	By choosing 2 or more postures and making a nice smooth transition between them, we create a meditative flow. We work the breath into the flow and allow the postures to move with our breath. For example: Starting in child's pose, exhale. Smoothly flowing to a cobra, inhale. Coming back through table top to a child's pose, exhale. We continue the flow imagining we are a wave breaking on the shore.
Trees	**Balances**	Tree pose: taking the weight on to one foot we raise the other up, placing it above or below the knee and bringing the hands to salutation at the chest, above the head, or opening the arms to make branches.
		We can also practice tree with a partner or with everyone in a circle. A **Drishti** is the still point we find to focus on.

Flowers	**Balances**	Standing one legged balances: dancers pose, half moon, folded binds, bird of paradise – there are many postures we can do on one leg, imagining we are a beautiful flower. (See website for resources.)
Animals	**Animal Postures**	We love to be animals! There are many postures in Yoga Asana where we get to be animals. In the jungle, at the farm, in the dessert. We can be a snake, a frog, a lizard, a horse, a cat, a camel, a cow. A theme can be chosen for your animal postures, maybe one week you are in Africa with lions and tigers and the next week you are in the garden, being butterflies and birds.
Homo-sapiens	**Warrior Postures and flows**	Here we can work on one specific posture or flow the warrior postures together. The most common warrior poses are: Warrior 1, 2 and 3, reverse warrior and humble warrior. It is fun to add in triangle or pyramid variations to help with the smoothness of the flow. (See website for resources.)

WARRIOR FLOW – STRONG AND STEADY!

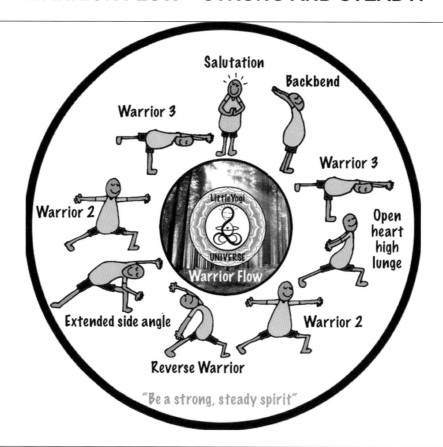

| Baby | Spine relaxing postures | When we are being a happy baby, we take an active posture to relax the spine, open the hips and re-center after moving our body so much. It is also nice to play in these postures as they are very safe. We can also take a rock and roll, giving ourselves a big hug and rolling backwards and forwards. |

Human	**Partner Work**	Partner work is wonderful, as we are now not only aware of our own body, strength, balance and breath, but also of an other's. When we do partner postures we feel connected through touch and physical support and we also should feel safe and have lots of fun! Partner yoga can be practiced with a parent and child, students in a classroom or peers in a yoga class!
Every one	**Sivasana**	A form of Yoga Nidra Meditation. Students lie down with their legs apart and arms away from the sides, palms facing up to the sky. In this position it is important the whole body is comfortable so that each muscle can relax completely and the mind can be free from thoughts of physical discomfort. In this posture there can be a guided meditation, a body scan, a mantra, silence etc. it is a time to fully relax and feel the connection with the self and the others in the room.

| Universe | Meditation on Union. | Once we have finished our Sivasana, we can take a little bit of time at the end of the class to sit silently and feel gratitude, compassion and union with ourselves, with others and with the universe. We feel thankful for our bodies and the people that love us and we say thank you to our parent, teacher and any others in the class for sharing the yoga practice by saying: **Namaste** "My soul honors your soul" or "My inner universe, honors your inner universe." |

For more resources and information visit:

www.littleyogiuniverse.com

Printed in Great Britain
by Amazon

64916386R00030